The Ultimate Smoothie

By Stephen T. Radentz

Disclaimer

I am not a doctor. I am not giving health advice. I am just giving you some basic facts about some very healthy plants. The information contained in this booklet is for general information and educational purposes only. It does not constitute medical advice. Therefore, any reliance you place on such information is strictly at your own risk. Please check with your medical doctor before starting or changing your medical routine.

Acknowledgments

A big thank you to my family for believing that my health was worth fighting for. Love you guys (Chris, Jake, and Matt).

THE ULTIMATE SMOOTHIE

Here it is the self-proclaimed, world famous smoothie that was the catalyst for healing my body after 50 years of abuse.

I was addicted to legal opioid pain relievers and nearly killed myself by making poor health choices. Finally, after being hospitalized with a corrosive bleeding ulcer, I decided that I needed to make some changes in my life. My first step was adding a variety of fruits, vegetables, herbs, and a couple of other secret ingredients to my morning routine. This allowed my body to begin healing, which in turn brought positivity to my mind. I began to be happy. There is a lot more to a perfectly balanced and happy life than the Ultimate Smoothie, however this smoothie can begin the process for you, too.

If you can say yes to any of the following questions, you may need to raise your nutrient intake at the start of the day.

- Do you feel tired or run down during the day?
- Does your energy level and positive attitude wane, and you don't know why?

- Do you find it difficult to stay positive in the morning, and by lunchtime, you are ready to unload on the next person who crosses your path?

It could be that you're not starting each day with a full tank of nutrients.

The first step on my journey to becoming synthetic-drug and processed-food free, healthy, and positive was to get my body right. I needed to detox 50 years of bad food, alcohol, and medicinal choices.

For Christmas, knowing that I was going to try to change my eating habits, my wife and sons bought me a NutriBullet. That gift began changing my life. I started drinking fruit smoothies every day. In a six-month period, I refined my "perfect ingredients," and then, for two months, I paid attention to how mixing up the ingredients changed how I felt during the day. During this time, I researched each ingredient, learning about how the plant grew, how the ingredient was processed or made, and the health and nutrient benefits. I wanted to know how I would benefit by consuming the ingredient and what negative side effects I could create (if any).

The items I use in this nutrient blast have been designed to create balance in my health and life. To this day, I still drink it at least three times a week. The combination of fruit, vegetables, herbal tea, and secret ingredients will blast your body with all the nutrients you need to start your day. You will feel more energized throughout the day. You will be able to accomplish more, have complete mental clarity and focus, and just feel better.

Let me say that this was and still is a perfect blend for *me*. If you don't like or can't eat some of the ingredients, feel free to mix it up. For instance, avocado is an amazing food that would also work in this mix. however, it's not my favorite flavor or texture. My only requirement is that you include the berries. I believe them to be one of the best cancer busters, and I feel that they should be eaten at least five times a week. Just my opinion; not scientific at all.

In the following pages you will find not only the smoothie ingredients but the health benefits of each one. I want you to understand how each nutrient will help you maintain homeostasis and good health.

Research is showing that knowing how nutrients work with our bodies can increase the healing process. It seems that having the expectation of known results multiplies the benefit. Your mind expects to receive a certain benefit and it knows how the nutrients should work in your body. This then increases the healing performance of the nutrients. I believe this is similar to the placebo effect. Our minds have impressive capabilities that we just don't know enough about.

For each ingredient, I tell you how its nutrients improve the three life centers (brain/head, chest, and gut). The reason for this is to show you that each ingredient is designed to balance your body as most natural foods accomplish this.

I smoked cigarettes for more than 40 years, so you might notice that I focus a lot on anticancer-type foods. I try to knock cancer cells (as I call them zombie cells) out of my body. I use that term because just as zombies can kill or transform you, a cancer cell can kill your good cells or transform them into cancer cells.

The cannabis community has adopted the phrase "whole plant medicine," which basically means you use all the ingredients in the plant as nature intended. I believe in using all parts of the plant or fruit to receive all the benefits. I do not recommend supplements, as they are only fragments of plants mixed to give your body a boost. Unlike synthesized supplements, which can cause unnatural side effects, whole plants (fruits, vegetables, herbs) not only give you a natural boost, but they also give you a balance boost that creates no unnatural negative side effects. Our bodies are designed to work with nature in a symbiotic way. Plants are designed to support the whole body, not just parts of it. If you want to have balanced health, use the whole plant.

Committing to this one food choice, the ultimate smoothie I began changing my life. I have learned that the first step to having a happy, healthy, abundant life is to *get your body right.* This blend of natural food can help you begin to do that.

It will take more than a smoothie every morning to achieve total balance, happiness, and abundance in your life. You will need to remain positive and grateful for life, and you will need to embrace nature in other ways as well. (Check out my other books for more ways to incorporate natural nutrients, and positivity into your life.)

The first two steps I took to leading a healthier life were drinking the Ultimate Smoothie and drinking 60 ounces of herbal tea every day. This ensures that your body starts the day with all the nutrients it needs, and then you replenish nutrients as the day goes along.

This smoothie recipe is a great starting point for good health. It is the recipe I used to begin eliminating pharmaceutical drugs and most processed foods from my diet. As I was learning how to live without deadly opioid pain relievers, this recipe gave my body the strength it needed to repair the damage I had caused. Today it gives me the ammunition my body needs to fight sickness. These foods are not the whole answer to good health; however, they will help your body and mind get moving in the right direction.

This smoothie recipe can help change your life. It changed mine, and it continues to benefit my mind and body. When you make a habit of filling your body's nutrient tank the first thing every day, you will begin to see improvement in other areas of your life. You can stop *trying* to improve your life and take the easy route and just eat better. Starting with the Ultimate Smoothie.

I know you are eager to get to the knock-out information in this booklet, so without further ado, here you go....

Smoothie Recipe

- 2 cups mixed berries (blueberries, blackberries, strawberries, raspberries)
- 1 carrot (or 4–6 cocktail carrots)
- 4-5 cherry tomatoes (or half a tomato)
- ¼ cup acai puree
- ½ –1 banana
- 1–2 large kale leaves or equivalent
- 1 kiwi
- 10 purple grapes (green or red are OK, too)
- 1 tbsp honey
- 1 tbsp apple cider vinegar
- 5 ml cannabis tincture
- 1 tsp bee pollen
- 10–15 oz herbal tea (mix it up)

Not everyone approves of the bee pollen, and I also have mixed feelings about it, but sometimes I add a teaspoon of bee pollen. It makes a noticeable difference in my energy level throughout the day.

If I feel a cold coming on, I add the juice from an orange, a quarter of an apple, and possibly some ginger.

,I currently use a three-speed blender, which works simply fine.

Once you've got everything in the blender, mix it on high for about a minute. You now have an amazing nutrient blast (approximately 28 ounces) for your body.

Now for the really cool part. Get ready to find out how these ingredients can improve your health and help you prevent or eliminate sickness.

Health Benefits

Blueberries

Blueberries are one of my favorite fruits. If you don't want to get cancer, eat them every day. These little berries, as well as blackberries, contain high amounts of anthocyanins, the chemicals that blast unwanted free radicals, which can cause cancer. Most purple fruits have anthocyanins that battle cancer cells. They are a great defense against disease.

They contain hefty amounts of vitamin C, coming in at 24 percent of the recommended daily amount, plus vitamin K at 36 percent and manganese at 25 percent. Blueberries also contain vitamin A (good for eyesight), iron, magnesium, and potassium. They're small but they pack a punch of nutrients.

You can find reasonably priced blueberries at most grocery stores all year. Feel free to buy them frozen if they aren't available fresh, as the frozen variety has just as many nutrients.

Here's a cool fruit hack: *Freeze blueberries at least 24 hours before eating them to make them super sweet. I've tried to figure out the science of why this happens and have come up empty handed, but frozen blueberries are sweeter than fresh.*

Here's how blueberries can help your three life centers (head, chest, and gut):

Head
- Improves memory and cognitive response
- Has antiaging properties
- May improve Alzheimer's disease and dementia symptoms
- Improves learning capabilities

Chest

- Improves circulation
- Improves lung function
- Improves immune system
- Reduces risk of cardiovascular disease
- Protects artery lining to ensure optimal blood flow through body

Gut

- Supports liver function to improve removal of toxins
- Improves kidney function
- Boosts immune system
- Supports digestion

Blueberries are one of a handful of fruits native to North America. Their use can be traced to the beginning of Native American history. A little-known fact about blueberries: they've been gathered in the wild for centuries but weren't commercially cultivated until the early 1900s. I'm so glad these little nutrient blasts are a commercial crop. I love them and try to eat them every day because I know their knock-out nutrients are healing my body.

Blackberries

Here is a fruit that will jump-start your health with cancer fighting anthocyanins' I love harvesting wild blackberries; it is so cool to pop them in your mouth out in nature. I love covering blueberries and blackberries with honey, heating them to make a sauce, and pouring the sauce over vanilla ice cream. So yummy, and helps your desert become healthier.

Blackberries are high in vitamin C (one cup has about 35 percent of the RDA), and they also have high amounts of vitamins K and A. They contain 14 percent of the RDA of fiber. Blackberries can prevent tumors, and they have anticancer properties due to their high antioxidant values. Not only are blackberries one of the best tasting berries (in my opinion), but they are also one of the most beneficial for your health. They are zombie-cell (free-radical) killers. As with most purple and blue produce, they contain high amounts of anthocyanins, which assist boosting the immune system while attacking cancerous or diseased cells.

Keep reading to find out how blackberries can help balance your life centers.

Head

- Boosts brain function
- Improves memory
- May improve or reduce symptoms of Alzheimer's disease and dementia
- Enhances mood
- Can reduce symptoms of depression

Chest

- Improves blood circulation and insulin response
- Reduces inflammation in arteries
- Increases lung function

Gut

- Reduces cholesterol
- Lowers stomach acid and improves digestion
- One cup contains 30 percent of daily fiber needs

Blackberries have been around since ancient times. The Greeks and Romans used the plant as a medicine and food source. The body of a well-preserved woman who lived more than 2,500 years ago was found with blackberries in her stomach. Just another treat that nature has provided since the beginning of time.

I feel that the biggest benefit of blackberries is that they are an incredible antioxidant. They are a powerhouse of nutrients. Now if we could just figure out how to keep the seeds from sticking in our teeth.

Raspberries

Low in calories, high in fiber, and loaded with vitamins and minerals, raspberries are also filled with micronutrients, phytonutrients, and anthocyanins. The raspberry has 53 percent of the RDA of vitamin C, as well as vitamins B6, K, and E, calcium, magnesium, iron, phosphorus, manganese, copper, lutein, lycopene, zeaxanthin, and potassium. This little berry is an excellent source of nutrients. Antioxidants are abundant, making them zombie-cell killers.

Head
- Improves cognitive functions
- May reduce symptoms of Alzheimer's disease and Parkinson's
- Reduces stress

Chest
- May reduce cardiovascular disease
- Reduces high blood pressure
- Anti-inflammatory

- May help alleviate symptoms of diabetes

Gut

- May help reduce obesity , by filling you up without the calories,
- Aids in digestion
- Promotes healthy bacteria growth in the gut

Raspberries are being studied for their anticancer benefits. The research findings are showing that, like other types of berries, eating them can reduce or eliminate cancer cells. If you're not including this tart fruit in your diet, you are missing out. Try them in a salad or soaked in a tea blend.

The raspberry has been used as a medicine and food source since before the time of Christ. Archeologists have found evidence of early humans using it. The Romans are thought to have been the first people to cultivate and popularize its use. In 1761, George Washington began cultivating raspberries in his extensive gardens. Native Americans harvested and dried the berries as an energy and medicine source during nomadic moves around the country.

Today the largest commercial raspberry farms are located on the west coast of the United States, where more than 70 million pounds are harvested every year.

Fruit Hack: the leaves of the raspberry plant can be used in tea and medicinal tinctures and used to treat digestive issues as well as menstrual cramps.

Strawberries

Strawberries are loaded with nutrients and antioxidants. The fruit contains vitamins A, C, K, calcium, potassium, magnesium, and iron. All of that and they're cholesterol free as well. Strawberries have been known to reduce inflammation and improve the symptoms of neurological disorders. One of the sweetest berries, they are great right off the vine When I was young, my family had a small patch in our backyard. Every morning during the summer I would go outside and harvest the fresh berries for the day. That is one of my earliest memories of me connecting with nature.

Nothing is better than picking and eating food right from the source.

Head
- Antiaging
- Improves cognitive function
- Improves memory and learning abilities

Chest

- Reduces inflammation
- Improves blood circulation
- Improves lung health

Gut

- Increases food bacteria growth
- Promotes healthy digestion
- Anticancer

Strawberries, like most berries, have been used for centuries. They have been referenced in writings and artifacts from Greece and Rome. In the 1500s strawberries began being cultivated for use as a food and medicine. Hippocrates could have been referring to a strawberry when he said, "Let food be thy medicine." Instructions for growing and harvesting strawberries first showed up in writing in 1578.

Here's a little-known fact: Strawberries and cream was created by Thomas Wolsey in the court of King Henry VIII.

Today in the United States, more than a million tons of strawberries are harvested each year. California produces the bulk of them, and Florida is in second place.

Plant City, Florida, has a strawberry festival in late February or early March. More than 500,000 visitors attend and eat strawberries in hundreds of different ways. I highly recommend you check it out someday!

Bananas

Who doesn't love bananas? I like mine in a smoothie (or banana split). They are another super beneficial fruit packed with nutrients. Bananas have 3 grams of fiber and 1.3 grams of protein. They contain vitamins A, B6, and C, magnesium, manganese, iron, copper, and potassium.

Bananas are known to protect against developing type 2 diabetes and reduce swelling. Another fruit loaded with antioxidants; another zombie-cell killer. In case you're wondering, overripe bananas contain more nutrients than green bananas.

Head
- Mood enhancer
- Antidepressant (releases serotonin)
- Improves focus
- Improves cognitive function

Chest
- Maintains proper blood pressure
- Improves blood circulation

- Assists in regulating the nervous system

Gut

- Promotes healthy liver and kidney function
- Reduces indigestion and heartburn
- Improves digestion
- Reduces or eliminates nausea

Eating a banana is a great way to eliminate nausea, as well as reduce cholesterol. If you are feeling nauseated, reach for a banana.

There is evidence that bananas were cultivated in the highlands of New Guinea at least 7,000 years ago, and that Musa varieties were being bred and grown in the Mekong Delta area of Southeast Asia as many as 10,000 years ago. That makes bananas one of the oldest known cultivated crops. Apparently, humans have always liked bananas. Sometime around 1500, they were brought to the Americas by Spanish missionaries. However, they were not a popular commercial item until the 1800s.

In case you were wondering, a banana tree can grow 10 feet tall in 4 months and produce its first fruit in about 6 months. I know people in colder climates who grow banana trees in large pots, and in the winter, bring them inside to keep as houseplants, making bananas available all year.

Bananas are especially great for your gut, but they'll also give you whole-body benefits. Enjoy one today.

Grapes

Grapes are another great nutrient bomb. Purple and red ones (like most purple and red fruits) are loaded with antioxidants and anthocyanins, which make them a great anticancer food. Green grapes are also loaded with nutrients.

Grapes make great wine, and some folks have claimed that a glass of wine every day is good for your heart. However, a group of Spanish scientists found that the benefit was from the *grapes,* not the wine. You no longer have a health excuse to drink wine. Sorry dudes and dudettes.

Grapes have also been around since the beginning of time. Egyptian hieroglyphics show that grapes were cultivated more than 8,000 years ago. The Bible mentions wine more than 200 times, and the first mention of grapes is in Genesis, the beginning of recorded history. The oldest known winery, found in Armenia, was built more than 4,000 years ago.

Grapes have been extremely popular for a long time. They can be found on every habitable continent, and they have been used by all cultures since the advent of human life.

Head

- Improves memory
- Aids in Alzheimer's disease prevention
- Increases oxygen to the brain
- Relieves stress
- Improves attention span

Chest

- Lowers blood pressure
- Aids in the prevention of heart disease
- Improves lining of arteries, which reduces blood clots
- Improves lung function

Gut

- Contains fiber, which aids in bowel function
- Antibacterial effects may improve digestion by promoting healthy bacteria growth in the stomach
- May reduce kidney disease
- Improves kidney and liver function

Grape juice, or should I say ice-cold grape juice with no sugar added, is one of my favorite drinks. A super-sweet natural drink, and the health benefits are off the charts. Just like other fruit, grapes have anticancer properties, so when they're available, they should be included in your diet several times a month.

Acai Berries

Wow, here is an antioxidant powerhouse. Acai berries have an incredible number of anthocyanins, which have antioxidant properties that decimate zombie cells. I preach that we should eat blueberries every day because of their antioxidant benefits. However, acai berries have four times the number of antioxidants. The antioxidant content of foods is typically measured by its oxygen radical absorbance capacity (ORAC) score. In the case of acai berries, 100 grams of frozen pulp has a score of 15,405, while the same number of blueberries has a score of 4,669. I should also mention that acai pulp has more benefits than the juice. I buy frozen pulp or puree packages that are perfect for one smoothie.

Known for their antioxidant benefits, acai berries also blast the three life centers with nutrients. There is a reason acai berries are considered a superfruit. They contain vitamins A, B1, 2, 3, C, and E, as well as calcium, magnesium, phosphorus, potassium, iron, zinc, copper, and manganese. Simply loaded with natural goodness.

Head

- Improves cognitive skills
- Improves and strengthens memory
- Boosts the immune system
- May reduce Alzheimer's disease and dementia symptoms

Chest

- Improves cardiovascular health
- Reduces risk of heart attack and stroke
- Regulates blood pressure
- May improve lung health

Gut

- Regulates cholesterol
- May assist in weight loss
- Aids in digestion
- Encourages good gut bacteria growth
- May prevent or reverse liver disease

That is just the short list of amazing health benefits you can receive from acai. You may be asking yourself, "Where does this super food come from?" To answer that, it is a Brazilian or

Amazonian rainforest staple. The local inhabitants regularly eat the fruit, soaked in water to soften the skin, and then pureed. The fruit does not store well and must be processed within 48 hours, which is why in the U.S. we have only frozen puree or powder.

Until the late 1990s, acai was mostly unheard of outside the Brazilian rainforest. Ryan and Jeremy Black, two brothers from southern California, and their friend Edmund Skanda began exporting it to the United States. They fell in love with the fruit while on a surfing vacation in Brazil. That is how acai berries became a superfood outside the rainforest.

I want you to sound totally educated when discussing acai berries, so you should know that the fruit is not actually a berry because it has a central seed. It is called a drupe. Now you'll sound incredibly smart when talking about the acai superfruit.

Kiwi

This tasty fruit from New Zealand by way of China is also known as the Chinese gooseberry. Its name comes from the fruit's similarity in appearance to the New Zealand national bird, the kiwi bird, which is also small, brown, and fuzzy. Bet you didn't know that, or this: the kiwi was not available commercially until the 1970s. Look at it now; it's a superfruit that you can usually find year-round.

Kiwis contain some major nutrients. Here's the short list: vitamins A, B6, C, E, and K, as well as calcium, magnesium, iron, phosphorus, potassium, and only 3 milligrams of sodium. The kiwi hits the three life centers with a powerful nutrition punch.

Head
- Repairs damaged DNA
- Improves cognitive development
- Improves memory
- Reduces stress by releasing serotonin

Chest
- Improves immune system
- Helps regulate blood pressure and blood sugar
- Reduces triglycerides (fat in blood cells)
- Fights heart disease

Gut

- Aids in digestion by speeding up the processing of proteins
- Balances alkalinity in the stomach
- Reduces heartburn and indigestion
- Removes toxins and reduces risk of kidney stones

One kiwi has more potassium than a banana. It tastes a little like a strawberry. I have a system for peeling a kiwi: If it is hard (not ripe), simply slice in half, then cut the peel away with a very sharp knife. If it's softer (riper), slice it in half, then use a teaspoon to scoop out the fruit. Remember to compost the peel because it makes a great soil additive. Kiwi makes an awesome addition to any salad; it also goes well with fish. Have you ever heard the saying, "Eat a kiwi every day and you will keep the doctor away?" Maybe that was about apples. However, both apples and kiwis are great for your health.

Carrots

Wow! Nearly 300 percent of the RDA of vitamin A. Two hundred percent of the actual vitamin, and another 100 percent is converted from the beta-carotene content. Vitamin A is great for the eyes. Most people do not realize that carrots are also an amazing anticancer food. Several studies show that the phytonutrients in carrots reduce the risk of a variety of cancers. As a matter of fact, beta-carotene has also been found to reduce the risk of lung cancer.

Carrots have what you need if you want to improve and maintain your eyesight. The super-high vitamin A content is responsible for the claim that eating carrots helps eyesight. Vitamin A combined with beta-carotene can help you maintain excellent vision.

Head

- Antiaging properties
- Improves memory and cognitive ability
- Slows or stops macular degeneration
- Improves eyesight

Chest

- Improves circulation
- Reduces heart disease
- Reduces risk of heart attack
- Lowers blood pressure
- Assists in regulating blood sugar
- Regulates cholesterol

Gut

- Aids in detoxing kidneys and liver
- Improves digestion
- Helps control weight gain
- Promotes good bacteria in the stomach

Carrots have been consumed for centuries, dating back some 3,000 years. It appears that they have been commercially cultivated since 900 AD, when they were found in archeological digs in Afghanistan and Iran. Who knew? The original (pre-1500s) carrots were mostly white and red. Over time, with selective breeding practices orange became the color of choice for consumers.

One cool thing about carrot colors is that they reveal health benefits. For example, an orange carrot is full of beta-carotene, a purple one is high in anthocyanins, red is high in lycopene (also anticancer), yellow has lutein (anticancer), and white is high in fiber.

Here's a little secret: carrots add sweetness to a smoothie or salad, and they have less than 3 grams of sugar.

Kale

Kale is one of the most nutrient-rich foods on the planet. For years, I was not a fan of the taste of kale, however I have learned that I can blend it with other foods to make it easier to eat. I can feel a definite difference (more alert, focused, energetic, and healthy) on mornings when I include kale in my smoothie.

It contains 1,000 percent of the RDA of vitamin K and more than 130 percent of the RDA of vitamins A and C. It supplies 10 percent of your calcium, potassium, and vitamin B6 needs. It provides 1–7 percent of magnesium and iron, as well as micronutrients and phytonutrients. kale is exploding with health benefits.

Kale has been cultivated for 6,000 years; its use has been documented in Greek and Roman texts. It is found on every habitable continent. However, it has not always been a staple in people's diets. An interesting fact about kale in the United States: until the 1990s, it was mostly used as a decorative ingredient. Then its nutrient benefits were let out of the bag, and *bam,* it became a superfood.

Today, kale can be found in American stores year-round and should be included in your diet. The mega nutrients are incredibly beneficial for your body. Kale comes to the game ready to play; it has a powerhouse of nutrient benefits.

Head

- Improves memory
- Reduces risk of Alzheimer's disease and Parkinson's
- Reduces stress
- Helps maintain homeostasis

Chest

- Anti-inflammatory, which helps reduce heart disease
- Improves circulation
- Removes plaque buildup in arteries
- Reduces risk of lung cancer
- Aids in respiratory system function

Gut

- Builds healthy bacteria in the stomach
- Aids in digestion
- Builds immune system

- Helps detoxify the liver
- Improves kidney function

Kale has been blamed for causing kidney stones, but recent studies show that this is inaccurate. Kale provides most of what a human body needs to survive. If you only eat one green food, this is it. But remember, a single plant will not keep you balanced and healthy. Variation and moderation are key.

Tomatoes

Lycopene, a strong antioxidant, is the stand-out nutrient in tomatoes, and tomatoes have a lot of it. According to the cancer research center, and other sources eating tomatoes can reduce the risk of cancer. I've also heard that eating tomatoes with olive oil weekly can prevent many cancers.

Tomatoes also contain a good amount of vitamins A, B6, C, and K, plus beta-carotene, magnesium, potassium, iron, and calcium. Tomatoes contain only 10 milligrams of sodium and 2.7 milligrams of sugar in a 4-ounce serving. I eat at least five cherry tomatoes or the equivalent every day. They are one of my favorite fruits to grow. There is nothing better than going out to your garden and grabbing some fresh ripened tomatoes that you grew yourself.

Head

- Reduces cognitive impairment
- Improves memory
- Helps prevent Alzheimer's disease and dementia
- Improves eyesight

Chest

- Aids respiratory system
- Increases blood circulation
- Regulates blood sugar (anti diabetes)
- Strengthens heart muscles

Gut

- Improves digestion
- Helps regulate bacteria in the stomach
- Improves liver and kidney function

Tomatoes have been around since the beginning of time, and it seems that the Aztec nation was the first to cultivate them, around 500 AD. From Central America tomatoes were transported to Spain and Italy, and eventually became a staple food for many cultures.

Fruit hack: if you grow your own tomatoes, you can taste their freshly picked flavor. Pick them in the morning. There is a noticeable difference in the flavor of morning-harvested fruit vs. the afternoon. Morning-harvested tomatoes have a sweeter, more vibrant flavor. Try it and see for yourself.

Honey

"Nature's magic sugar substitute:" that's my name for honey.

The oldest known use of honey seems to be around 8,000 years ago. Cave drawings show humans harvesting it. A fossil of a honeybee dating back about 35 million years was found in Europe. We can assume that humans knew about honey for as long as we've been humans.

Honey has been used as medicine by most, if not all, cultures. The Babylonians, Egyptians, Assyrians, Greeks, and Romans (you know, the great civilizations of ancient history) all used it for its healing power. It has been used as a gift to God's being used in sacrifices. It has been used as wedding gifts between nations to bring families and their countries together., as well as a peace offering between rival nomadic tribes.

Humanity has been on the honey bandwagon since Adam and Eve. Many religions view it as a gift from God. It has been mentioned in the Bible 61 times. It was considered sacred to the Egyptians, and only royalty and spiritual leaders were allowed to have it. It has been used as an embalming fluid and found in tombs with pharaohs. With all this documented use, there must be something pretty special about honey.

The health benefits of honey are being researched. We are discovering the truth that the ancients knew thousands of years ago. Honey is an amazing anti-inflammatory, antioxidant, antiviral, and antibacterial agent. Its uses seem limitless; just do an Internet search. I will touch on just a few of the benefits.

Honey can support good dental health. The antibacterial agents in honey can reduce the bacteria in your mouth, which can reduce cavities. Imagine that. Honey, an all-natural sugar substitute, can aid in cavity prevention. Moms and dads let your kids have some honey after dinner; it will clean their mouths with sweetness.

Here's a fascinating fact: Honey contains an enzyme that, when combined with salt and a high-pH liquid (think sweat or blood) turns into hydrogen peroxide. What does hydrogen peroxide do? Sanitizes, sterilizes, and kills bad bacteria. But honey can only make hydrogen peroxide in the right environments; it works naturally with the human body. The ancients knew that it heals wounds, and twenty-first-century science is proving it.

I use honey every day; I eat it, it is also an ingredient in a health lotion I use for moisturizing my skin. Sometimes I will use it to help heal a scratch. I believe it is part of the puzzle of perfect health and balance. I believe it helps my body and mind reach homeostasis. According to one group of researchers, honey has more than 200 active micronutrients that benefit the body and mind.

It is not a coincidence that honey is the perfect sweetener. Nature makes it with zero help from humans. It has so many health and hygiene benefits. It is more than just a superfood.

I hope you can see that nature really does work with us, and in return we need to work with nature.

Let's look at the three life centers and how honey can help you reach homeostasis.

Head
- Improves memory and cognitive function
- Improves brain development
- Reduces stress
- improves sleep

Chest

- Reduces risk of heart disease
- increases blood circulation
- Reduces coughs and sore throats
- Improves respiratory system
- Improves lung function

Gut

- Promotes healthy digestion
- Promotes good bacteria growth in your gut
- Helps prevent liver and kidney damage
- Has prebiotic properties

Honey hack: When you heat honey to 98 degrees, you begin killing many of its nutrients. If you want to cook with honey and get all the amazing benefits, let your recipe cool down first, then add the honey.

One controversial claim about honey is that it can help prevent allergies. Many people swear by honey's ability to fight allergies, so maybe there's something to it. The theory is that because bees collect an assortment of pollen, if you eat local honey, you raise your immunity to local pollen. The key is that you must eat locally harvested honey because local bees make honey from local plants—the ones affecting your allergies. Except that bees collect pollen mostly from *flowers,* while allergies stem from *grass and tree pollen,* not flower pollen. Regardless, it might work, and it won't kill you, so why not try it?

When buying local honey, the general guideline is to look for a raw, unfiltered, and uncooked version. If the label says it's pasteurized, it has been cooked and many of the benefits have evaporated.

Honey has been a staple in humans' lives for millennia, and I believe its healing abilities speak for themselves. It's a strong natural medicine for many ailments. It's no wonder that bees protect their stores so fiercely.

Apple Cider Vinegar

There are very few nutrients in apple cider vinegar (ACV for short). It contains about 11 milligrams of potassium, 1 milligram of sodium, and less than 1 milligram of sugar per tablespoon, and carbs. Zero protein, or calories. Yet it has an amazing way of healing.

I'll compare it with rain and plants. Rain basically contains zero nutrients, but when it rains, plants grow like crazy. ACV, like nature, just has a mysterious power when people use it, according to their testimonies they tend to be healed. Do a Web search on "ACV healing benefits" and you will find thousands of health claims?

When I started consuming ACV, I noticed that I felt better, I digested food better, and (gross, I know) my hemorrhoids stopped bleeding. I changed nothing else in my life when I started taking ACV. My diet had been much improved over the previous year, and I had all but stopped drinking alcohol well before I learned about it. But I believe it triggered a healing effect in me, and, just like that, the hemorrhoids improved. Just so we're clear, I consumed the ACV; I did not use it topically.

Apple cider vinegar has antifungal, antibacterial, antiviral, and antimicrobial properties. You could also use it as a topical scrub, and it would clean you up. You can use it to disinfect surfaces. I have used it to knock down weeds in my garden. (All vinegar is acidic; you must be careful around some plants.) It can also be used in homemade bug spray. It is pretty amazing stuff.

Head
- Improves mood
- May elevate serotonin levels, which promotes happiness
- Increases cognitive function

Chest
- Regulates blood sugar
- Helps maintain a healthy cardiovascular system
- May reduce risk of heart disease

Gut
- Promotes and maintains healthy bacteria
- Improves liver and kidney function
- Increases nutrient absorption
- Promotes weight loss

Apple cider vinegar is not a miracle cure-all formula. It does seem to have the healing power people are looking for. I suggest that you try a teaspoon once a day. I add a tablespoon to my daily smoothie, and I miss that vinegar taste when I don't add it.

To start using ACV, focus on one area of your body that needs healing and see what happens. Always mix ACV with water or juice. You can even cook with it to get your daily dose. Note: ACV has high acid content and could upset your stomach or create heartburn issues, so start slow.

When buying ACV, look for an all-natural or organic version "with the mother." The mother is the yeast and bacteria used to create it. You are looking for unrefined, unpasteurized, and unfiltered apple cider vinegar. As with most products, when it gets refined and pasteurized, it loses many of its nutrient benefits.

I take ACV almost every day. When I don't, I can feel the difference. It may all just be the placebo effect, and I'm OK with that. In my opinion, apple cider vinegar is an all-natural medicinal product, whether or not science proves it. If it works and it doesn't kill you, go for it.

Cannabis

What if I were to tell you that cannabis and hemp, to a smaller degree, are superfoods?

Many people say, "I don't want anything to do with that nasty marijuana; I don't want to feel high." Well, let me tell you one simple truth about cannabis. Unless you heat marijuana to above 215 degrees, you will not get high. Heating THCA and CBDA activates the chemicals into what we know as CBD and THC, which we normally associate with cannabis. When eating cannabis or hemp in its natural raw state, you get a plethora of nutrients for good health, and you will not get high.

Secondly, there are at least 17 vitamins and minerals, including magnesium, calcium, phosphorous, , beta-carotene, potassium, sulfur, iron, zinc, vitamins C, B1, B3, B6, and E. It also contains protein, carbohydrates, insoluble fiber, as well as more than 100 cannabinoids that help create homeostasis in our bodies. Cannabis is loaded with phytonutrients, micronutrients, terpenes, fiber, essential oils, and the perfect ratio of Omega 3, 6, and 9 and more (a 3-1-1 ratio is the perfect omega balance for humans).

The health benefits of raw, whole-plant cannabis rival kale, which is one of the most nutritional plants on earth. That makes cannabis one of the most nutritious plants on the planet. It is a superfood in its raw state.

Head

- Relieves stress
- Releases serotonin
- Improves cognitive function
- May reduce Alzheimer's disease and Parkinson's symptoms

Chest

- May improve lung function
- Relaxes blood pressure
- Promotes healthy heart function
- High in antioxidants

Gut

- Relieves nausea
- Improves digestion
- Improves liver and kidney function

Cannabis has been used since the beginning of time. Every ancient culture has archeological evidence of hemp and marijuana use, as well as the cultivation of the plants. Hemp oil may be mentioned as kaneh-bosm in the Bible in Exodus 30: 22-23 (second book, in the beginning). Hemp was found in the pyramids. Every farmer in America and England was required to grow hemp because of its many benefits. Even after prohibition, during the second world war, in 1942-1944, hemp could be grown to make rope to support the war effort.

Cannabis and hemp are amazing plants with amazing benefits for our health. To find out more simple truths about marijuana, check out my book Medical Marijuana: The Simple Truth.

CONCLUSION

There you have it. One amazing, life-changing, immune system–boosting, happiness-making smoothie.

I spent most of my life eating processed foods and consuming excessive amounts of alcohol and social drugs. Entire years went by in which I didn't eat fruit or vegetables. When I decided I needed to change my diet and life, this smoothie recipe is what began making my body healthy and balanced again. This exact formula was my first step to a balanced life.

You have no excuses for not starting your day in a healthy way. Feel free to substitute items. However, I suggest that you research the ingredients first. As I said in the beginning, you can increase the impact of natural nutrients by understanding how they will benefit you and your body.

My wish is that you will have a long, healthy, and happy life. I know that natural foods can impact your life in a most positive way. Begin with this smoothie recipe in the morning to get your day started, and then add some herbal tea blends to bolster your health throughout the day. These are two of the easiest ways to attain great health. If you're anything like I was, eating healthy must be easy and convenient, or forget about it. Making a smoothie or a half gallon of herb tea is simple, and anyone can do it.

Eat and medicate naturally, maintain positive momentum, be grateful, and embrace nature. That is how you become balanced by nature. It's how you can start easily living a balanced, healthy, happy, and abundant life.

Speaking Engagements

Stephen is available to share his journey and insights with your organization.

For more information, contact him at Steve@balancedbynature.net

Stay up to date on his thoughts on life at Balancedbynature.net.

If you enjoyed this booklet, check out 2 of my other plant health booklets.

- Five Herbal Tea Recipes to Balance Your Life
- Medical Marijuana: The Simple Truth